This Curly Woman Went Gray

Pamela Cummins

Copyright © 2022 by Pamela Cummins

All rights reserved. No part of this publication may be reproduced, distributed, or transmitted in any form or by any means, including photocopying, recording, or other electronic or mechanical methods, without the prior written permission of the publisher, except with brief quotations embodied in critical reviews and certain other noncommercial uses permitted by copyright law.

ISBN-13: 978-0-9976703-5-6

Cover Designed by Brent Meske

Book Formatted by Triomarketers

May you embrace your beautiful gray hair and enjoy the freedom to be who you are!

Contents

Why I Stopped Dyeing My Hair 1

Three Paths to Gray Hair 9

Transition Beginnings 19

Advice for Curly Hair 31

Polite Hair Trolls 41

Heal Your Hair Story 55

Conclusion 65

References 67

About the Author 71

More Books by Pamela Cummins 73

Why I Stopped Dyeing My Hair

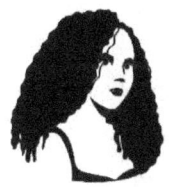

I was never a girly girl; instead, I preferred the natural look and never bothered with straightening my hair or using makeup. The idea of dyeing my hair didn't occur to me either. When I was twenty-five, someone pointed out my first gray hair and yanked it out to show me. I felt embarrassed, yet I had no intention of ever dyeing my hair.

In my early thirties, the front of my hair turned silver, and it didn't bother me. Although my gray hair annoyed other people and, boy, were they vocal about it! One of my colleague's customers kept harping on me to dye my hair because I was too pretty to go gray. I dated a man who told me that my garlic breath turned him off, that I needed to cover up my gray hair, and since I didn't have sex with him by the third date - the relationship was going nowhere. We never had a fourth date and I still eat food with garlic and other yummy spices.

After many people pestered me, I caved and allowed my hairstylist to cover up the grays. Thus began the vicious hair dyeing cycle that lasted for over twenty-five years...

Inspiration to Stop Painting My Hair

In May 2020, during the Covid lockdown, I had the following dream:

In my dream, my hairstylist of seven years had died from Covid-19. I became very upset because I care about her. Also, who else could do my mop as well as she did?

Then in the next dream scene, I was angry at a male hairdresser and arguing with him because he wouldn't listen to how I wanted my hair done. Instead, he kept telling me how my hair needed to be.

Upon awakening, I was worried that my hairstylist had died and hoped she was okay. Her salon was closed during the Covid lockdown and I hadn't heard from her since my last dye job on March 11, 2020. Because I've been interpreting dreams since the early 90s, I knew how precognitive dreams felt, and this dream was in some way related to my future. What a relief when I got a text from my hairstylist and she was alive.

Before, during, and after reading my hairstylist's text that her salon was now open, I kept hearing my angel whispering *no* over and over.

I sent her a text to ask what the mask regulations were at the salon. Her response was she would let her clients decide. My decision was to listen to my angel. So, I didn't schedule an appointment.

My precognitive dream meaning was guiding me to let go of my hairdresser and find another one. It was also a warning of how the hair industry and much of our patriarchal society are against women going gray. Additionally, I would need to deal with these hair trolls.

Fast Forward to Today

It's been over two years since I had my hair painted and will continue for at least another year. Or I might have the ends cut off when I turn sixty. What an amazing journey it has been! My hair is so healthy and I'm in love with it! Another benefit of this experience is it enhanced my personal and spiritual growth.

To assist with my transition, I was a member of a video online support group for three months, and joined and participated in gray/silver Facebook groups. I have spent countless hours reading books and researching the internet for information about transitioning to gray and the best methods for curly hair. This research was the reason I chose the cold turkey method to transition to my natural hair color. You'll learn more about going cold turkey in the next chapter.

My expertise is dream interpretation, spirituality, and personal growth; I am not an expert on hair. However, I learned to listen to my angels' guidance because it's always right; hence, the reason for writing this eBook. My wish for those reading this eBook is to pass on all the knowledge I have learned and to share my experience about my curly hair transition from dye to salt and pepper hair.

I suspect you are reading this book because you have your own concerns about transitioning to gray hair, and I hope you find something

This Curly Woman Went Gray

of value here. Please take what you want and leave the rest behind.

Three Paths to Gray Hair

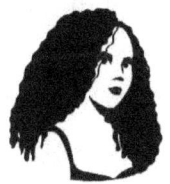

Congratulations, you have decided to stop the everlasting process of using hair dye! Your hair will thank you by becoming healthier and healthier. There are three paths to transition to your natural hair color.

1. Cold turkey and letting your hair grow is the longest path.

2. The chop to a short haircut is the quickest.
3. Lowlights, highlights, and other techniques done at a hair salon to help blend your grays better with the dyed hair color.

Let's go over each technique, which works for all hair textures.

The Chop

Cutting your hair into a pixie, bob, or another style will quicken the process of growing to your gray hair. A chop removes most or all of the dyed job. If you like your hair short and the way you look, then this would be the best path for you.

Curly hair women can look gorgeous with short hair, especially those with a thin density.

However, if you prefer your hair long or have thick, coarse, curly hair, then this isn't the best route. I grew out my short hair to long hair at the ages of six and twelve. Yuck, it was a nightmare! My hair grows out like a mushroom top. On a good hair day, it looked like Bozo the Clown with Shirley Temple curls. And forget about it on a bad hair day, my hair was even worse!

Hair grows on an average of a half inch (1.27 cm) a month. Yours may grow slower or faster. The school of thought for hair growth is in one year it grows to your ears and in two years it will reach your shoulders. Except curly hair shrinks anywhere from two to twelve inches (5.08 to 30.48 cm). For instance, if your curly hair is shoulder length, it can shrink below or above the ears. And if you have my hair texture, it will grow sideways.

Longer hair can mellow out the thickness and stretch out the curls.

Salon Techniques

Another way to transition is to have a salon do lowlights, highlights, toning, and other techniques. Women with lighter color hair can have luck with these hair treatments. Nonetheless, you are playing Russian roulette with your hair.

Three Paths to Gray Hair

Victims of playing Russian roulette tend to be women with darker hair from these salon treatments. Their hair can turn green or orange causing some to dye their hair again. Others had their hair fried, which could result in hair breakage, and being forced to cut their hair shorter. The dryer your hair, the more damage can happen. Curly hair tends to be dryer because the oil from the scalp can't travel smoothly down the hair shaft as it does with straight hair. Also, these salon techniques may ruin your curls.

For those who choose to go this route, it is very expensive and demands a ton of upkeep to maintain healthy hair. I don't know about

This Curly Woman Went Gray

you, but I stopped painting my hair to save time and money, plus I wanted to avoid chemicals seeping into my scalp and brain.

Two warnings about transitioning gray hair with this route.

1. Don't allow just any colorist to perform these techniques on your curly hair; instead, search for an expert. Then ask for references with pictures and talk to these women before scheduling an appointment.

2. Please don't try this on your own. An impatient woman with black dyed, curly hair bleached it several times. She

ended up destroying her curls, having a weird blonde color, and cutting it above her ears because her hair was so damaged.

Cold Turkey

Going cold turkey is the longest way to go gray, especially with long hair. It sometimes feels like it's taking forever. I have no regrets taking this route, although some people thought I was crazy to transition my hair this way. These are six benefits of going gray cold turkey:

1. You can have the hair length you want, whether that's short, to your shoulder, or down to your butt.

2. There's no risk of damaging your hair.

3. You will spend less money at the salon.

4. You'll have more free time because of fewer salon visits.

5. This helps you to ease into and become used to viewing yourself with silver hair.

6. If you despise the way you look with gray hair, you can dye it again. More importantly, you didn't lose your length or waste money on blending or other salon treat-ments.

Letting your grays emerge cold turkey takes courage, yet it's worth the benefits. My suggestion is to test it out for at least three to six months. You can always try the other two paths later.

Transition Beginnings

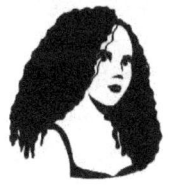

When you first stop covering up your grays, it can be compared to stopping smoking or giving up sugar; it's difficult and feels uncomfortable. You may wonder if everyone is looking at your gray demarcation line thinking that you can't afford a dye job, are unkempt, or being lazy.

This Curly Woman Went Gray

Ladies, your skunk line is your badge of honor, welcoming change and a new way of life.

In the beginning, some of you might question whether this is the true color of your gray. In all likelihood, it's not your actual color. Why? When your demarcation line is only a few inches, it's too small to determine the color. Your silver hair will pick up the tone of your dyed hair; therefore, the color could change when all of the painted hair is gone. Lighting will also affect the color of your hair. Your silver will become lighter in the sun and under bright lights, while darker in the shade and lower light settings.

Transition Beginnings

My natural hair color today looks totally different than it did at three months dye free. Thicker hair is a benefit that I and other women receive when they stop the hair dye. It was shocking for me to see how many baby hairs sprouted out in the beginning for me. I like to think the new growth was my hair thanking me for letting it be itself.

Another thing I like to point out is that your natural hair color might be white, silver, steel, salt and pepper, salt and cinnamon... Many of us have more gray in the front, while the back and underneath are a darker color. Whatever your natural hair color is, it's unique and beautiful, which beats any boring dye color.

Helpful Tips

There's a silver revolution going on as more and more women are kicking the dye habit. You are not alone on this journey. The following tips helped me and may help you.

Find Support

Your family, friends, coworkers, and others might not support you; especially in the beginning when your skunk line is showing. Even strangers might have something to say. You will learn more about this in the chapter about polite hair trolls.

It's imperative that you find support. Luckily for you, there's a ton of support from Facebook groups, Instagram accounts, and other social media platforms to assist you during your transition. A few of these groups are for curly women only. Most of these groups are supportive and helpful with information. Social media being what it is, I've encountered a few unpleasant women and one judgmental group. I blocked the women and left the group. Only stay connected with women and groups that are helpful.

What I found inspiring was viewing before and after pictures of women who went from dye to their natural hair color. In my opinion, these women *looked better in the after pictures.* Their silver hair caused their complexion to glow and look healthier. In fact, I discovered that most of these ladies appeared younger. Imagine that - gray hair didn't age them!

Research

Knowledge is power. You're reading my eBook, yet I want to encourage you to read other books about transitioning to gray hair. Explore the internet for the wealth of articles, blogs, and videos on this topic. Also, if you find someone's information confusing, then continue to research it.

Hair Accessories

Hair accessories are a great way to cover up the demarcation line when you go out in public. Here are seven ideas:

1. Baseball caps
2. Hats
3. Turbans
4. Scarves
5. Headbands
6. Wigs
7. Hair extensions

Temporary Color

Some women use root spray or a temporary color while transitioning.

Others have fun with colors of blue, green, pink, and more. A word of caution – make sure you use a coloring product that *washes out* in one to five shampoos. Semi-permanent color can stain your grays, so only use it on the dye part of your hair.

Hairstylist

Sadly, your hairstylist may not be supportive of you stopping the dye. They may tell you, "It will age you. You're too young to go gray. Or you will hate it." Your stylist might truly believe what they are saying, since the hair and beauty marketing campaigns have influenced our society. Or perhaps he/she is afraid of the loss of money they make from you every month?

Please don't allow your hairstylist to talk you into dyeing your hair. This goes for what type of hairstyle you should have, too. You are PAYING them to do **what you want**, not what they desire. Sadly, you may have to fire them if they continue to make snide comments or do not give you excellent service. My hairdresser of seven years kept putting LOL in the texts she sent to me upon finding out I was letting my gray come in. Her LOL, energy behind the text, and lack of mask enforcement caused me to seek a replacement. I am thrilled with my new hairstylist! Her salon is closer to my home, she uses healthy products on my hair, and most important of all, she listens to what I say and cuts it the way I ask her to.

If you need to find a new stylist, read the salon reviews. Always listen to your gut. If a salon feels off, go with the one that feels right. Then I would suggest calling the salon and asking if they are *gray and curly hair friendly*. If they are, schedule an appointment. Before you put your butt in the chair, tell your hairstylist what you want, and ask them to repeat it back to avoid miscommunication problems. If at any time, your intuition is warning you something is not right; clarify what you said or leave.

Special Events

At six months dye free, I wore my long, curly hair in a braid to officiate my niece and her fiancé at their big, fancy wedding. If I can do that, you can also go to a special event with multi-color hair. Wear a fancy hat or hairstyle. There's no need to dye your hair for one day, no matter what a polite hair troll says.

Keep Going

This journey isn't easy. Gray groups and supportive gray friends are the places to go when you feel like caving and dyeing your hair. *This too shall pass* and you'll be grateful that you didn't dye your hair. Think about the time and money you have saved. Your *future self* will thank you for going through the moments of struggle and how beautiful your hair is without the paint.

Advice for Curly Hair

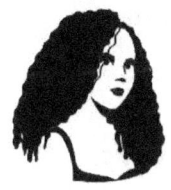

This chapter's advice is useful for wavy, curly, and kinky hair; however, in each of these categories, what works for one person may not work for you. My suggestion is to research and learn about your hair type. The following four categories are important for you to know:

1. Discover if your hair density is thin, medium, or thick.
2. Find out if your hair texture is fine, medium, or coarse.
3. Learn whether you have low, medium, or high porosity hair.
4. Research your curl type that begins with 2A wavy hair and ends at 4C for kinky hair.

Are you wondering why bother and what does it matter anyhow? This will assist you with how often you need to wash your hair, the best way to style it, and find hair products that work for you. Many curly hair women have tested a bunch of products to find *the one* that works best for them, which cost them a fortune. There are even curly hair groups where they trade their barely used hair products. By learning your hair type, you will quickly find the right ingredients for your hair type; saving you time, and money.

For example, most of my curls are 2C and 3A with some 2/3B mixed in. It's also thick, coarse, and has low porosity. I wash my hair every five to seven days. Scrunching my hair works best for me, although sometimes I'll finger curl my 2B hair. Products that work best for me have lighter ingredients; for instance, aloe, argan oil, and jojoba oil. Many curly girl products contain shea butter, coconut oil, and heavy proteins, which my hair won't absorb, instead the product lies on top of it, and looks awful. Hence, I avoid hair products that contain those ingredients. I have saved time and a lot of money by not experimenting with the wrong shampoos, conditioners, and so forth.

Whatever types of hair products you use, it's important to avoid sulfates, silicones, and parabens. What I discovered is that expensive organic and salon products actually save you money. How? You will use smaller amounts of these products because there is a higher percentage of quality ingredients, while drugstore products use fillers.

Another hint I have to avoid hair damage/loss when using a new product is to test them on your pubic hair; a good reason to not completely wax or shave it off. Wouldn't you prefer hair damage or loss down there instead of on the top of your head?

You might want to read the book *Curly Girl the Handbook* by Lorraine Massey, and there are now many variations on it. Avoid falling down the curly hole by reading the mega amount of articles and watching videos, as I have spent time there hour upon hour for months and months. Watch out for the Curly Hair Police who will belittle you for not following it to their specifications.

You may have no desire to find out your hair types or to research curly hair methods. Whatever you choose to do, here are eight tips I learned that will make a world of difference for your hair:

1. Wash your hair less to avoid stripping out the oils. When cleansing your hair with shampoo or co-wash, focus on your scalp area, while using very little on the rest of your strands.

2. Use conditioner on every washday, but avoid your

scalp as it produces its own oil.

3. Detangle your knots with your fingers, wet brush, or a wide-tooth comb ONLY when your hair is wet and slathered with a lot of conditioner in the shower or over a sink. For easier detangling, start at the bottom while working your way to the top. The only time you brush or comb your hair dry is when you want wild hair to go with a Halloween costume.

4. Apply leave-in products and style your hair when it's wet.

5. Use a cotton t-shirt instead of a towel to avoid frizz and for better looking curls.

6. Avoid heating tools; air dry hair to prevent yellowing your silvers and having the texture of dry leaves. If you must dry your hair quickly, use a diffuser hair dryer.

7. Sleep on a silk or satin pillowcase for less frizz and tangles.

8. Put your hair in a silk bonnet, or gather it up in a pineapple (ponytail like Pebbles on the Flintstones) before going to bed. This will preserve your beautiful curls.

Advice for Curly Hair

Those eight suggestions may at first seem overwhelming and very time-consuming. It took me a while to get used to it, yet I'm glad I did because my hair is healthier and looks so much better. Test out some of these techniques to see if they work for you, even if it's just using a cotton t-shirt instead of a towel.

Gray hair can become yellow from the sun, hard water, heating tools, and more... Hats and umbrellas are useful for protecting your hair color. A water purifier helps with hard water. Some women use blue and purple shampoo, which I never bothered with. Silver hair yellowing is another topic for you to investigate.

A word about frizz – *Frizz Happens*. I've learned to embrace the frizz, especially since I live in North Carolina, USA, where the humidity can reach a hundred percent during the early mornings of summer. Even Andie MacDowell has frizz and she probably has an entire staff of people who work on her hair for celebrity events. Frizz gives your hair personality.

Polite Hair Trolls

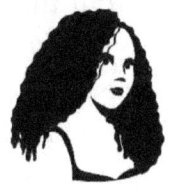

A stranger approached me as I was washing my hands in the ladies' room. "You have beautiful curly hair," she said. I thanked her for her compliment. Then she informed me she was a hairstylist and how she would straighten my hair, thin it out, put highlights in it, and cut it short. Wait? What just happened? I was in a state of shock, replied how my hairdresser would kill her, and walked away.

This was only one example of unsolicited advice from the thousands I received. Every curly woman has dealt with someone who gives an unwanted opinion about their hair. Their advice may cause you confusion or feel as intrusive as a salesperson calling at midnight. Sometimes you can laugh at the advice and forget about it. Other times, their words hurt, and bring tears to your eyes.

When a curly woman receives unsolicited advice about her hair, it goes beyond the words. You are picking

Polite Hair Trolls

up on their tone of voice, their energy, and the intention behind the advice. You feel their anger, jealousy, and other emotions. Then you have to deal with your own feelings and wonder how to respond to their unwanted opinion. This can be overwhelming.

Thankfully, I have supportive loved ones during my silver journey. My mate told me how relieved he was that I stopped using chemicals on my head. Then there are other people who I wished had kept their mouths shut. Women in my gray groups have written about the harsh words they received. Hence, I came up with the phrase *Polite Hair Trolls*.

Four Types of Unsolicited Advice

Not all unsolicited advice is equal. This advice can range from polite to downright insulting. The four types of unsolicited advice are:

1. Rude Advice
2. What You Should Do
3. Compliment, Then Critique
4. Their Experience

To help you identify the four types, I'll go over each one, using three examples, and why the person gives their unwanted advice.

Rude Advice

Some people don't use filters with their words. Or they hide behind their computers and leave rude comments on the internet. Here are three examples of rude advice:

1. Gray hair makes you look old.
2. You look like a witch with that hairstyle.
3. You're too little to have all that hair, you need to cut it short.

Usually, rude advice is from insecure people. They criticize others to feel better about themselves. You need to consider the source on whether there is any truth to their words. Do NOT discuss this issue with the rude person, even if there is an element of truth to what they are saying or writing. Instead, find somebody who is safe and supportive to discuss the issue with.

What You Should Do

This type of advice isn't as rude, yet who are they to *should* on you? Their recommendation about how to improve your appearance is a roundabout way of them being judgmental. If you're hurt by their words, they hide behind, "You're so sensitive," "I'm just being helpful," or "It's for your own good." The three what you should do are:

Polite Hair Trolls

1. Don't go cold turkey growing out your gray hair, you should get highlights done.
2. You should straighten your curls.
3. I think you would look better with short hair, you should cut it.

Perhaps this person has your best interest in mind. What a shame they didn't ask for your permission to share their advice and/or word it differently. Sometimes, you will ponder their words over and over, while feeling hurt. Please listen to your intuition and logic on whether or not their advice is worthwhile for you.

Compliment, Then Critique

Do you remember the stranger who told me I had beautiful hair and how she would change everything about it? Yup, she complimented me, then critiqued me. It also has a flavor of *what you should do*. Here are three examples of compliments, then critique:

1. Your curly hair is so pretty, why don't you perm it to have your curls lay better.

2. I like your natural hair color, there are products that will brighten up the gray.

3. Your hair transition looks great. You could totally get away with a chop, maybe some layers, too.

Why someone compliments, then critique you is because they're insecure, jealous, or are making themselves seem superior to you. It's confusing because what they first said made you feel so good. And then you got sucker punched. Allow yourself to acknowledge what truly happened and why you feel the way you do.

Their Experience

This one is the trickiest out of all four types of unsolicited advice. They aren't rude or telling you what you should do. Instead, they are telling what works well for them. However, if this is the case, why does it feel so yucky or judgmental to you? Because you're picking up their energy of unsolicited advice that can have a critical and/or a superior vibration to it. The three examples of their experience are:

1. I find coconut oil makes my hair so nice, I bet it will help you with your hair.

2. I straighten my hair because I can't stand so many different curl types as they stare at your curls.

3. When I went gray, I got highlights because I couldn't stand the brown ends. Going cold turkey must have been a hard two years for you.

Although people's experiences may have been right for them, this doesn't mean it will work for you. Create your own experiences on what is right for you.

How to Deal with the Four Types of Unsolicited Advice

Now that you know what the four types of unsolicited advice are, it's time to go into how to deal with it. Here are ten suggestions:

1. Ignore rude advice, even if they press your buttons again to get a reaction.

2. Delete their comments and / or block them on social media.

3. Block that person on your phone.
4. Talk to someone in HR if this is a work-related issue.
5. Walk away from opinionated strangers.
6. Choose silence as a response.
7. Respond, "Opinions vary."
8. Let them know this topic is not up for discussion.
9. Quote Bernard Williams, "Unsolicited advice is the junk mail of life."
10. Journal down what happened to release your thoughts and feelings about the incident.

Polite Hair Trolls

Keep in mind that most people's intentions are to be helpful when giving advice and they don't mean to hurt you. Yet others want to harm you with their words. If you're dealing with a bully and feel physically threatened; keep silent, walk away, or call for help.

Please don't give unsolicited advice. Think about what your intentions are with the advice. Are you coming from a place of love? Or are you judging them? What are you feeling at the moment? Would this advice benefit their life or situation? Lastly, always ask for their permission first to find out if they're open to advice.

Heal Your Hair Story

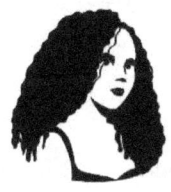

Everyone on the planet Earth has lessons to learn that happen during our life experiences. Some of those experiences can cause issues and trauma, which each individual needs to heal. Many think that denying their feelings and forgetting about an awful event won't have any consequences; nonetheless, they do NOT disappear as they remain stuck in our body, mind, and spirit. As a healer, I've experienced, learned how to, and assisted my clients to heal those memories and emotions stored in our bodies. Yet it never occurred to me how hair also holds onto trauma and issues, duh. Maybe it's stored within the roots?

Full confession time; all those examples of unsolicited advice are from my experiences. The remark, "You're too little to have all that hair. You need to cut it short," was a comment made by some random female customer. This happened over thirty years ago at my former job in a men's clothing store. Obviously, I didn't respond to her comment because at the time I needed to be professional at work. Her words made me feel hurt and very uncomfortable, so I stuffed those feelings and memory down until decades later when I began the journey of returning to my natural hair color.

Curly hair females (and men) receive a ton of comments and unsolicited advice. Folks with straight hair do not know what curly women go through. Often, our caretakers were clueless about how to take care of our curly hair. I have a horrible memory (at eight-years-old) of my grandmother tugging and ripping through the knots on my dry hair with a brush, while cursing my mother for allowing it to get that tangled.

For years, most beauty schools didn't teach how to cut and style curly hair. Hairstylists would insist on straightening, thinning out, doing razor cuts, or using heating tools. Thus, causing hair damage and even more frizz. This caused many of us to have haircut trauma. I remember fantasizing about throwing a brick through a hair salon's window after a horrendous haircut. This was decades before online reviews.

Hallelujah! There are more curly hair schools and salons than ever before. Women are not only embracing their true hair color, they are accepting and showing off their natural hair texture. All hair texture is beautiful, and it's important to accept yours.

When you're on the path of growing out the dye, it's imperative to review and heal your personal hair story. You could have flashbacks or nighttime dreams about your hair trauma. Or experience heightened emotions about your hair without knowing the cause. One time I wanted to rip off a polite hair troll's head. Now what they said was inappropriate, but my emotions and reaction to their comment were extreme. Thankfully, I didn't act on it;

instead, I realized my feelings were being magnified from similar past experiences.

Suggestions to Heal Your Hair Story

Even if you are not having heightened emotions, nighttime dreams, or flashbacks about your hair; I encourage you to examine your hair history. The following seven suggestions can aid you:

1. Write/type, voice or video record, or visualize events pertaining to your hair.

2. Take notice of what feelings come up while you're recording these events.

Heal Your Hair Story

3. Release the feelings by feeling them, whether it is anger, sadness, confusion... It may help to write, speak, or visualize at the same time as embracing past emotions. Hug a teddy bear while the tears flow. Or visualize throwing balls of healing light at those who angered and hurt you.

4. Do sessions with a coach, therapist, or spiritual adviser to help you through the process.

5. Forgive yourself and others ONLY when you are ready.

6. Promise your curly hair that you will always protect it.

7. Tell yourself and your hair how beautiful they are, even on a bad hair day.

Relapse Dreams

Alcoholics and drug addicts aren't the only ones who have dreams of relapsing. Women have dreams about dyeing their hair. Upon awakening, they can feel devastated about the idea of having to start their gray journey all over, then feel relieved it was only a dream.

These hair dye dreams occur to keep us on track with our journey. And reveal our genuine emotions about our former dyeing practice. Therefore, these dreams are healing dreams, even though they are uncomfortable.

Sometimes women have relapse dreams on their dye free anniversary: one month, six months, one year, five years, or ten years after the last paint job.

Healing From the Inside and Out

So there you have it. This journey not only heals your hair and financial status, you're also healing emotions and feelings from your hair story.

Perhaps you think I am foolish for having this chapter while revealing parts of my hair story. Or you're wondering if you should bother dealing with your hair story. The reason to heal from your hair story is you'll increase your self-confidence and become empowered. I know this happened to me and my hope is it will happen to you.

Conclusion

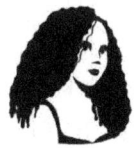

In my Facebook silver hair groups, women have written *it's only hair, it will grow*. If that was true, then why does the hair industry earn billions upon billions of dollars each year? How come we spend so much time and money on our hair? If it is only hair, why do we cry over a bad haircut or loss of hair from health issues?

It's more than hair! Besides protecting our scalps, it's our identity. Hair strands enhance our face. Like Samson, our hair signifies our power. Hence, the reason to take care of it and love it.

Even if you only take one of all the suggestions in this eBook, my work is done. Honestly, I hope you adopt more than one of the recommendations. Ignore the polite hair trolls and heal your hair story. Embrace your gray, curly hair and don't care what others think. It's your hair and it's your choice of what to do on your hair journey...

May you have many good hair days!

Blessings,
Pamela Cummins

References

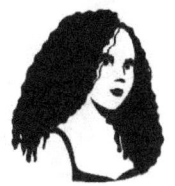

This section has my favorite resources to help with your additional research. All the links work at this time, but I can't guarantee they will work in the future.

Books

Silver Hair: Say Goodbye to the Dye and Let Your Natural Light Shine

by Lorraine Massey

This Curly Woman Went Gray

Going Gray: What I Learned about Beauty, Sex, Work, Motherhood, Authenticity, and Everything Else That Really Matters

by Anne Kreamer

The ABCs: How to Always Be Curly and Love It!

By Adina Sherman

Websites

Katie Goes Platinum
https://katiegoesplatinum.com/

This Organic Girl
https://thisorganicgirl.com/

Naturally Curly
https://www.naturallycurly.com/

Frizz Forecast (this is from the Naturally Curly website and is very useful)
https://www.naturallycurly.com/frizz-forecast

Facebook Groups

The following are private groups:

Curly Silvers
https://www.facebook.com/groups/1943436612549095

Silver Revolution (Group by Katie Goes Platinum)
https://www.facebook.com/groups/silverrevolution

The Gray Book – Inspiration for Going Gray (Group by This Organic

Girl)
https://www.facebook.com/groups/thegraybook

About the Author

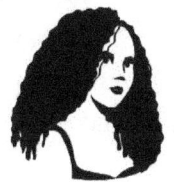

Besides Pamela Cummins being a gray curly woman, she is an expert dream interpreter and spiritual growth intuitive. Pamela is the author of books on the topics of dream interpretation, personal growth, spirituality, and relationships. She also writes two blogs. In her free time, she spends time with the love of her life, a spoiled princess kitty, and a parakeet who tweets and tweets and... Pamela reads one or more books a week, enjoys yoga, and going for walks. Learn more about her at: https://www.pamelacummins.com/ and https://learndreaminterpretation.com/

More Books by Pamela Cummins

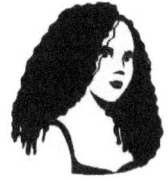

The following books are available on many eBooks platforms. You can find the links to your favorite eBook store and country you live in here https://books2read.com/Pamela-Cummins

This Curly Woman Went Gray

Learn the Secret Language of Dreams

Do you know that your dreams are special and unique? But if you don't understand their meaning, you are missing out on vital information. Because every night your subconscious mind sends you messages to help you solve problems, improve relationships, and teach you how to create a higher quality of life. The key is to learn how to decipher them and that is how Pamela Cummins, dream and relationship expert, can help you. *Learn the Secret Language of Dreams* is designed to give you the ability to understand the meanings of your own dreams.

Symbolism in dreams is not a "one size fits all." One symbol can mean many things. In order to understand the nature of dream symbolism more clearly, you will need to know what category your dream fits into. This book will help you identify the different dream styles so you can recognize what part of your life the dream message is for. Once you know the category of your dream, it will be easier to interpret your unique personal symbolism.

Personal Growth Affirmations

Do you desire more happiness and peace in your daily living? Did you know that you can have the life you always dreamed of? Change is possible; however, all transition starts within. *Personal Growth Affirmations* will motivate you to begin the process of your transformation journey with fifty-two weekly affirmations to be used for self-help and/or meditation.

Some of the topics are: self-love, forgiveness, patience, gratitude, boundaries, meditation, connecting with a Higher Source, the ups and downs of living, and much more. The affirmations have questions to inspire reflection, action steps to help you transcend, and a short mantra to be chanted any time you feel the need. Manifestation of your aspirations becomes reality by applying the wisdom of each affirmation. Now is the time to start your journey...

Insights for Singles: Steps to Find Everlasting Love

Insights for Singles: Steps to Find Everlasting Love delivers insights to help readers reach their highest potential, learn to think positively, recognize red flags, how to let go of a relationship, improve communication skills, and understand how to *attract* and proceed with the "Right One." Whether you need to learn to "Keep your pants on" or "My fantasy is not reality," singles will find plenty of *potent* insight and *proven* solutions in this book.

This Curly Woman Went Gray

Psychic Wisdom on Love and Relationships

Do feel like you will always be single? Are you sick of bad dates and relationships? Bored and unsatisfied in your relationship? *Psychic Wisdom on Love and Relationships* is a unique book packed with wisdom for BIG relationships. Go inside the world of a psychic to see how the spirit world gives knowledge to transform your love life. This book will take you on the journey of self-love, boundaries, intuition, communication skills, and more.

More Books by Pamela Cummins

Got Dreams? Discover Your Ideal Dream Journal

Have you ever told yourself upon awakening that you will remember the dream you just had, but forgot large chunks of it within minutes? This is why it's imperative to record your dreams. Yet, what journal style would work best for you?

Expert dream interpreter, Pamela Cummins, has your answer and more. In *Got Dreams? Discover Your Ideal Dream Journal*, you will learn: nine different types of dream journals, the benefits of journaling your dreams, how dream interpretation will empower your life, and a glimpse into understanding your dream meanings.

Pamela's Love Collection

What do self-love, the *Three F's*, and "He has to be spiritual" have in common? They are all in *Pamela's Love Collection*. Love is always in the air, but often it's just out of our grasp. It is time to start grasping it whether you are single or in a relationship. You will learn how to recognize the signs of healthy love and what to do with it. This eBook consists of twelve articles, blogs, and columns by love intuitive and radio host Pamela Cummins.

www.ingramcontent.com/pod-product-compliance
Lightning Source LLC
Chambersburg PA
CBHW020302030426
42336CB00010B/865